DMT: The Truth About Dimethyltryptamine

The Ultimate Beginner's Guide to a Revolutionary Compound and Its Full Effects

Table Of Contents

Introduction

Chapter 1: What Is Dimethyltryptamine?

Chapter 2: History of Dimethyltryptamine

Chapter 3: The Science Behind DMT

Chapter 4: The Effects of DMT

Chapter 5: Pros and Cons of DMT

Chapter 6: DMT Compared to Similar Substances

Chapter 7: The Future of Dimethyltryptamine

Conclusion

Introduction

You've probably heard about DMT some time before. Maybe you've heard about how it is supposed to give people who consume it some semblance of euphoria, or how it can somehow alter one's way of thinking. So what exactly is DMT, also known as Dimethyltryptamine?

Well, in this short and concise book, we will get into the history of DMT, recent developments that involve the substance, the science behind Dimethyltryptamine, the potential future legalization, and how the compound can affect one's body. Most practically, we will also look at the pros and cons of this compound and how it compares to other similar "drugs", especially the short-term and long-term effects of consumption.

In this book we are aiming to look at this topic in an unbiased light. We are not promoting the consumption of DMT, per se, but we want to make sure that if someone is interested in this controversial topic, he or she can reach more informed conclusions.

We hope that you are able to learn a thing or two!

Chapter 1:

What Is Dimethyltryptamine?

Dimethyltryptamine (DMT), which is part of the tryptamine family, is a psychedelic drug that is naturally occurring. This substance naturally occurs in the human body and in certain plants. In the human body, DMT is created during normal metabolism by serotonin (a neurotransmitter) and tryptamine-N-methyltransferase (an enzyme). Through consumption, the substance can be inhaled, injected, or ingested. In the natural world, DMT can be found in several different plant species with genera, including virola, piptadenia, mimosa, acacia, and many others.

Richard Strassman was one of the first psychologists to study DMT and other psychedelic substances' effects. Dr. Strassman discovered that dimethyltryptamine is released by the pineal gland when a person nears death. This discovery potentially explains why people who go through near death experiences often report vivid imagery, or NDE (near-death experience) phenomena. Interestingly, the substance is also released during day 49 of fetal development. Dr. Strassman attributes this to the soul's beginning. The substance is most often referred as the "spirit molecule" or "God molecule."

Uses of DMT

In its various forms, many cultures and ethnic tribes all over the world, particularly in South America, use dimethyltryptamine. During cultural rituals, ethnic tribes use DMT to be spiritually connected with God. South American tribes inhale and ingest yopo (anadenanthera peregrina) - a plant that contains a considerable amount of DMT. Ingesting or inhaling the substance can lead one to experience psychedelic episodes.

Amazonian Amerindian tribes also ingest the substance by consuming ayahuasca (an entheogenic brew) for healing and divination purposes. In the United States, many people use vaporizers and bongs to inhale DMT. The substance's effects last for only a few minutes, but the "high" one experiences while consuming DMT is completely state altering and considered intense.

Dangers and Effects of DMT

In a nutshell, when taken in excess and indiscriminately, dimethyltryptamine can pose a life-threatening health risk. Users of DMT can go into a drug-induced coma or reach an unconscious state. Oftentimes, unconscious users may start to vomit, thus leading to choking and death.

When consumed in moderate doses, the various possible effects of using DMT include increased body temperature, increased heart rate, lung irritation, overwhelming fear, stomach discomfort, altered concept of time, and intense psychedelic visuals. Other possible effects include hallucinations and feelings of movement or time slowing down or speeding up. Colors may become distorted and one could experience double vision.

The Law

In many countries, dimethyltryptamine is considered a Class A or Schedule I drug. This means that it is illegal to possess, sell, or give away to others. For possession of DMT, the maximum penalty is seven years jail time and/or a large fine. Even if one supplies or gives away DMT, even to friends, one risks landing in jail for life or, at the very least, paying a huge fine.

If one is caught by the police when using or possessing DMT, the police usually take action, including a formal caution, prosecution, or arrest. The implications are serious if one is convicted for a drug-related offense. It can disallow one from entering other countries and the types of jobs one can apply for are limited. It is also illegal to drive while one is under the influence of DMT.

Taking DMT

The substance is not orally-active unless it is combined with an MAOI (monoamine oxidase inhibitor), like those found in harmala alkaloids, which are produced by plants such as the ayahuasca vine (*Banisteriopsis caapi*) and Syrian rue (*Peganum harmala*). In the human body and with no inhibitor, monoamine oxidase rapidly breaks down the DMT that has been orally ingested and there is none to minimal psychoactive effects. In its pure form, DMT is normally smoked or injected.

Chapter 2:

History of Dimethyltryptamine

In 1931, Richard Manske attempted to synthesize dimethyltryptamine during a major wave of chemical experimentation following mescaline's discovery at the end of the 19th century. During that time, neither DMT's effect on human consciousness nor the substance's prevalence in South American tribal concoctions were known, so DMT was forgotten until a few years later when the South American shamans' potions and mixtures became the subject of interest in the blossoming field of psychopharmacology.

In his 1946 publication in Spanish, O. Goncalves first isolated dimethyltryptamine from *M. teniflora* (*Mimosa hostilis*). After that, more investigations from the South American shamans' plants resulted in

DMT being isolated later from both *P. Peregrina* and *Piptadenia macrocarpa*. That was in 1955. Despite its considerable use by cultural tribes in South America, the general public did not find out DMT's psychoactive effects until Stephen Szara reported it in 1956.

Szara, a Hungarian psychiatrist and chemist working from behind the Iron Curtain, was unable to acquire mescaline or LSD from Sandoz. Thus, he synthesized his own DMT after he had read about the substance's presence in South American shamans' plants. He then hoped that he would discover "psychedelic" properties in his synthesized substance.

After unsuccessful oral doses, Szara concluded that a gastrointestinal system enzyme or substance might be neutralizing the dimethyltryptamine. Szara became the first person to find out DMT's psychedelic properties when he self-injected the synthesized substance. His eventual research would publicize dimethyltryptamine to the world.

Shortly afterwards, Szara and his DMT stash fled from Hungary and then migrated to the U.S. where he found work at Bethesda, Maryland's National

Institutes of Health. He proceeded to work there for more than 30 years. Before he retired in 1991, Szara was the National Institute on Drug Abuse's Director of Preclinical Research.

Illegal Substance

In 1966, dimethyltryptamine was declared illegal after the substance was introduced in the fledgling psychedelic underground through the writing correspondences of Ralph Metzner, Timothy Leary, and William S. Burroughs. Burroughs had written to Leary that DMT was dangerous for experimentation after he almost overdosed while self-injecting it in London during 1960.

Nick Sands is credited as finding out that DMT could be smoked, wherein the discovery had briefly increased DMT's popularity among underground users. In 1968, Agurell, Lindgren, and Holmstedt first deduced that ayahuasca's effects were a result of the combination of naturally occurring DMT and monoamine oxidase inhibitors.

In 1970, the United States Congress passed the "Scheduling Laws," which made it almost impossible to research DMT, LSD, and mescaline in the country. Congress's ruling stopped scientific research into DMT within the United States until the FDA-approved clinical trials of Rick Strassman at the University of New Mexico. These trials took place from 1990 to 1995.

While DMT was (and still is) illegal in the United States, other international governments allowed its use to some degree and research on DMT continued internationally. The likelihood that dimethyltryptamine could be endogenous to human beings first came to light after scientific researchers found DMT in rats' and mice's brains. In 1965, a German team stated that they had derived DMT from human blood.

In 1972, Julian Axelrod discovered that DMT was found in the brain tissue of human beings. He subsequently found DMT in human urine and in fluid (cerebrospinal) that bathes and surrounds the brain. As the pathways by which the body made DMT were found out, the substance was declared the first endogenous human psychedelic. In 1965, S. T. Christian found 5-MeO-DMT in cerebrospinal fluid.

Chapter 3:

The Science Behind DMT

DMT (dimethyltryptamine) is a member of the tryptamine compound family that comprises of biologically-active compounds, including neurotransmitters such as the main pineal hormone and 5-hydroxytryptamine (serotonin), entheogens and melatonin, including DMT, 5-HO-DMT (bufotenine), O-phosophoryl-4-HO-DMT (psilocybin), and 5-methoxy-dimethyltryptamine (5-MeO-DMT). All these compounds have a similar indole-ring structure, wherein the indole backbone can be considered a portion of the structure of more complicated entheogens like ibogaine and LSD.

The Indole Ring

While magic mushrooms (psilocybin) and LSD are two of the best-known psychedelic tryptamines, the tryptamines of particular interest are the endogenous entheogens like 5-MeO-DMT and DMT. Why are they interesting? This is because the two entheogens do not have to be laboratory-manufactured nor are they extracted from a toad's venom or a plant. The substances are produced somewhere within the human body. Because they are endogenous, this means that they are really a part of the human system like bones, hair, or teeth are part of the human system.

As DMT and 5-MeO-DMT have similar structures as neurotransmitters, they can cross the blood-brain barrier and it allows them to have an intense effect on the human consciousness. DMT is especially unique as it is deemed a "brain hormone."

Neurotransmitters and Endorphins

While they can affect perception of spirituality and consciousness, dimethyltryptamine and 5-MeO-DMT are the only two entheogens that are naturally produced in the human body. The body is also known to create other familiar "drugs" like endorphins, which are morphine-like compounds.

The discovery of endorphins in the human body was deemed a major scientific breakthrough, and the people who discovered endorphins, for their efforts, were awarded the Nobel Prize. Many would think that discovering entheogens that are naturally produced would have been thought of as equally important. However, because of the oppressive measures that were burdened on the known psychedelics in the 1970s, research on entheogens was banned and progress was stunted.

Research on known psychedelics, like LSD and psilocybin, has gradually resumed over the years, particularly in regards to the substances' supposed medical benefits. The U.S. Drug Enforcement

Agency approved only one study on DMT. This study was the aforementioned University of New Mexico study conducted by Dr. Strassman between 1990 and 1995.

The Most Basic Tryptamine Psychedelic

Of all the tryptamine psychedelics, DMT is the simplest. Dimethyltryptamine, as compared to other molecules, is quite small and its weight is at 188 molecular units. This means that it is not much larger than glucose, which is the simplest of all sugars found in the body. Glucose weighs 180 molecular units, and it is 10 times heavier than a molecule of water (18 molecular units). For reference, the weights of other psychoactive substances are 211 molecular units for mescaline and 323 molecular units for LSD.

Dimethyltryptamine is a close relative of serotonin, and DMT's pharmacology is similar to other known psychedelics. DMT affects serotonin receptor sites in a similar manner to that of mescaline, psilocybin, and LSD. The serotonin receptors are all over the body and can be found in the skin, glands, muscles, and blood vessels.

The brain, however, is where dimethyltryptamine exerts its most dramatic effects. The sites that are rich in DMT-sensitive serotonin receptors are involved in thought, perception, and mood. While the brain blocks access to most chemicals and drugs, the brain takes a "special interest" when it comes to DMT.

Furthermore, a highly sensitive organ like the brain is susceptible to metabolic imbalances and toxins. The blood-brain barrier, which is a shield that cannot be penetrated, prevents "unwelcome" agents from leaving the bloodstream and transferring to the brain tissue through the walls of the capillaries. Such defense includes blocking the fats and complex carbohydrates that the other tissues utilize for energy. Instead, the brain burns glucose, which is the purest fuel form.

A few molecules, however, go through active transport across the blood-brain barrier. Some specialized molecules carry them to the brain, which is a process that requires a lot of energy. It is clear why, in many cases, the brain transports certain compounds into its territory. For example, amino acids that are needed to maintain protein in the brain can enter.

In recent years, DMT has enjoyed resurgence in the public consciousness. One can hope that more positive research will be done on both dimethyltryptamine and 5-MeO-DMT's unique properties.

Chapter 4:

The Effects of DMT

The restrictions regarding dimethyltryptamine usage and distribution vary from country to country. According to international law, DMT is considered a Schedule I drug under the United Nations' 1971 Convention on Psychotropic Substances, meaning that DMT's use is meant to be restricted for medical use and scientific research. However, natural materials with DMT (like ayahuasca) are not regulated under the Psychotropic Convention.

Generally, DMT is not addictive. A study on ritual users of ayahuasca concluded that, "A decoction of harmala alkaloids and DMT used for spiritual purposes has a safety margin comparable to methadone, mescaline, or codeine. Oral DMT's dependence potential and the dangers of sustained psychological disturbance are rather minimal.

Dr. Rick Strassman has recorded some of the physical effects of DMT. In his "Dose-response study of N,N-dimethyltryptamine in humans," Strassman recorded that a moderate dose of DMT led to a slightly-elevated heart rate, blood pressure, rectal pleasure, and pupil diameter. This is in addition to raising blood concentrations of corticotropin, beta-endorphin, prolactin, and cortisol. In his DMT study, Strassman noted that growth hormone blood levels equally rose in response to the DMT doses. Unaffected were melatonin doses.

DMT is not as addictive as alcohol, heroin, or cocaine, as dimethyltryptamine does not produce the other substances' drug-seeking compulsive behavior. Like addictive drugs, though, DMT produces increased tolerance in certain users who repeatedly take the drug. Such users then need to ingest higher DMT doses in order to achieve the results that they experienced in the past because of their built up tolerance.

Dimethyltryptamine is generally injected, smoked, or sniffed, and its effects are known as a "trip," which typically lasts for only 45 minutes to one hour. As mentioned earlier, when taken orally, DMT has no effect unless the substance is combined with other drugs. When taken in excess, DMT also comes with its own dangers. It can cause irrational judgment that leads to accidents and rash decisions. Excessive dosage can also cause frightening flashbacks or trips.

Major Effects of Dimethyltryptamine

It has been established that there are no long-term side effects of dimethyltryptamine, as the effects of using the substance last for, at the most, one hour. The psychedelic effects experienced while consuming the substance are largely based on the individual's subconscious mind. To such end, dimethyltryptamine can be dangerous, especially to users who have suffered mental health problems in the past. It is also not unheard of for users to have a bad trip and end up harming themselves in their state of panic.

Users will experience auditory and visual hallucinations, possibly with a euphoric feeling. DMT may change the user's perception of time's passage, wherein time seems to slow down or speed up. During this process, it is common for the pupils to dilate. As for the visual effects, most users agree that it is virtually impossible to describe what one sees to another person who has no experience with the drug.

As DMT can be adverse to people with a history of mental trouble, it can also be dangerous for people who enter a trip in a nervous or anxious state. DMT can also trigger the onset of latent or previously undetected mental health issues in some users. For some, the feelings of disquiet and anxiety can be amplified greatly during a trip. This results in a truly harrowing and terrifying experience that is usually accompanied with nausea and vomiting.

Users who have indiscriminately used DMT have been known to cause harm to others and to themselves. In such cases, there is a likelihood of suicide. Once a person starts tripping, there is no way to stop the trip until the effects diminish. This is why it is recommended by users to always have a sober friend with you if you are going to try DMT, especially for the first time. While there are some reported side effects to consuming DMT, flashbacks to bad trips have been reported by some users even after the drug's effects have worn off.

Psychological Side Effects of Taking DMT

Aside from the physical side effects of taking dimethyltryptamine, the psychological effects can be unpleasant for a user who does not know how to properly dose and consume DMT. Some of these psychological side effects can include depersonalization, emotional disturbances, realistic hallucinations, and spiritual emergency.

Spiritual Emergency

In a spiritual emergency, the psychological effects of DMT and other psychoactive drugs can be unsettling. According to psychiatrist David Lukoff, such experiences can lead to changes in reality's nature, which bring on anxiety and panic. A sudden change or loss in meaning is called a religious or spiritual problem, often referred to as a spiritual emergency.

Particularly, ayahuasca ceremonies can facilitate such occasionally painful ordeals in a cultural shamanic setting by combining DMT-containing substance use with other rituals like chanting. The ayahuasca tourism industry, which is gaining popularity, does not often help people who may experience psychological destabilization beyond the ceremony's confines.

Realistic Hallucinations

When it comes to realistic hallucinations, users who take psychedelics usually know that the hallucinations they experience are unreal, as they combine with one's sense impressions. However, when it comes to DMT, such knowledge does not necessarily exist. With DMT's dissociative effects, users can feel as if they are in another world or in a reality that is more compelling and vivid than waking awareness or dreams. According to the Office of Diversion Control, there are some DMT users who report altered an body image and realistic auditory hallucinations.

Emotional Disturbances

Under DMT's influence, many users may feel relaxation. There are also users who feel apprehension and fear, particularly if they are not comfortable with control loss during the trip's most powerful stage. In a 1994 study co-authored by Rick Strassman, there were reports of subjects experienced in taking psychoactive drugs who still felt that euphoria coexisted or alternated with anxiety. As with other tryptamines, DMT is not linked with addiction.

Depersonalization

Dimethyltryptamine, like other substances with tryptamine such as psilopcybe mushrooms, can lead to changes in how users identify themselves. Dimethyltryptamine metabolizes quickly and peaks in 90 seconds. This jumpstarts psychological shifts that the U.S. Drug Enforcement Agency has called the "businessman's trip." Absolute loss of identification and self with inanimate objects may happen and can lead users to experience deep existential thoughts.

Signs of Addiction and Treatment

While not addictive by itself, repeated use of DMT can lead to psychological addiction. This is where a user enjoys the drug's effects so much that he or she feels they can no longer function well without it. A user of DMT who is tripping is quite identifiable, as that user can hear or see things that are not real. A sign that someone is psychologically addicted to DMT is through irrational behavior on the user's part.

DMT is not a social drug, and a possible indication of DMT abuse can be spending more time alone and not responding to another person. The presence of hazardous materials and chemistry equipment may be a sign that a person is producing DMT for personal or commercial purposes.

Perhaps the best treatment to reverse DMT's effects is to engage in activities that are not drug-related. While DMT's effects are extreme, in theory, it should be more straightforward to give it up entirely. While recovering from a DMT addiction should not need too much medical intervention, it would be wise for a person to ask a doctor for advice in dealing with potential psychological urges that may occur.

Chapter 5:

Pros and Cons of DMT

The line that divides the positive points and negative points of dimethyltryptamine is somewhat blurred, with DMT being a controlled Schedule I or Grade A substance when artificially produced and being an unregulated substance when it occurs naturally in particular plants. The major issue when it comes to DMT is its legalization, in which the positive and negative sides present their points.

The side that opts for dimethyltryptamine's legalization has several good points. For several centuries, DMT has been used by various South American cultures as a tool for rite of passage, sacrament, or worship. The regulating of the substance in certain countries is what prohibits people from practicing their beliefs. Secondly, its psychedelic effects have been tested in regards to giving insight into one's self to fight off strong psychological processes like addiction. Moreover, the argument that dimethyltryptamine is "natural" because it is produced by the brain posits the point that one should be allowed to increase the natural amount within the human body, similar to how humans can add exogenous hormones.

Those who are against the legalization of DMT also present valid points. The substance is hallucinogenic, and when not used properly, DMT can lead to the endangerment of self and to others. Secondly, an MAOI (monoamine oxidase inhibitor) is present for the substance to be effective in oral brews with DMT. If used incorrectly, MAOIs can seriously harm the person and a bad tripping experience could psychologically scar a person for a long time. There are also studies suggesting that prolonged and/or overdosed DMT use is connected to schizophrenia.

Near-Death Experience

As mentioned earlier, the compound of dimethyltryptamine is linked to what is called a "near-death experience." In trying to resolve the near-death experience mystery, researchers have mentioned various theories on the possible causes. One of these theories is Carl Sagan's hypothesis through oxygen deprivation, neurochemical theories, and psychological dissociation. When it comes to neurochemical theories, psychedelic substances like DMT and ketamine have been implicated.

In Dr. Rick Strassman's book *DMT: The Spirit Molecule*, suggested that after one dies, the pineal tissue that starts to decompose might empty dimethyltryptamine directly into the spinal fluid. This allows the brain's emotional and sensory centers to cause residual awareness. D.R. Hill and Michael Persinger have also conjectured that all types of mystical experiences (NDEs included) might be from instances that trigger DMT's release from the pineal gland. Pim van Lommel, an NDE researcher, has written about the similarities of NDE and DMT trips.

However, there are also others who refute DMT's role in NDEs. Methodist University's Dr. Michael Potts compared the DMT experiences' elements with elements of an NDE present on the "NDE Scale" that was established by Dr. Bruce Greyson. According to Dr. Potts, key or frequent NDE phenomena have not been reported among DMT users, like traveling through a tunnel to reach another realm. According to him, permanent changes post-NDE apparently are the rule and not the exception, while permanent changes post-DMT experiences are more exception than the rule. Furthermore, Potts suggests that DMT is not the only substance that leads to the occurrence of NDEs.

The Most Powerful Psychedelic

Dimethyltryptamine is considered the most powerful psychedelic known to mankind. It is hard to ask research subjects to describe their DMT trip because most cases are intense. Additionally, they are often too difficult to process at the time for those who are new to the tripping experience.

Lastly, a dimethyltryptamine trip develops rapidly and lasts for only a short duration (one hour at most), but most trips can vary greatly depending on the individual, even if the setting is exactly same (unlike most psychedelics).

Chapter 6:

DMT Compared to Similar Substances

As dimethyltryptamine is a hallucinogenic substance, it is similar to and often compared to substances like psilocybin, peyote, ayahuasca, and LSD. All of these hallucinogens produce perception-altering effects by acting on the brain's neural circuits that use serotonin (a neurotransmitter). Particularly, some of the major effects occur in the brain's prefrontal cortex and other regions vital for regulating psychological and arousal responses to panic and stress.

However, the short-term effects of the various psychoactive compounds can vary substantially. In LSD, some of the effects include sleeplessness and dizziness. One may also experience sweating, dry mouth, and loss of appetite. LSD also increases blood pressure, body temperature, and heart rate. One can also experience tremors, weakness, and numbness. Users of LSD can also experience rapid emotional shifts and bouts of impulsiveness. Such shifts can range from euphoria to fear. There are also transitions that are so rapid that the user can feel various unexpected emotions at once.

Peyote is a naturally occurring substance, and it is found in a particular cactus native to Mexico and is being cultivated in parts of Texas. The substance, while controlled, is not as restricted as DMT. When taken excessively, peyote can result in flushing, profound sweating, ataxia, or uncoordinated movements, and increased heart rate and body temperature.

Psilocybin can occur in the form of what is often referred to as "magic mushrooms." When taking this psychedelic, users can experience feelings of relaxations (a similar effect when taking marijuana sparingly). Users can also experience spiritual/introspective experiences coupled with panic attacks, paranoia, and nervousness. However, the misidentification of poisonous mushrooms that look similar to psilocybin may lead to potentially fatal yet unintentional poisoning.

As for DMT, some of the effects include agitation, increased heart rate, hallucinations that always involve altered environments, as well as spatial and body distortions. As a derivative of DMT, ayahuasca can cause users to experience increased blood pressure and severe vomiting, which is tea-induced. When taking ayahuasca, one can also experience a state of shifted awareness and otherworldly imagery perception.

Effects of Hallucinogens

Whether they are manufactured, naturally derived from cacti or mushrooms, or produced naturally in the human body, hallucinogens, when taken excessively, do pose several intense and possibly dangerous effects.

Ingesting the hallucinogens can cause users to hear sounds, see images, and feel emotions that are actually unreal but seem real at the moment. The effects of hallucinogens typically take effect 20 to 90 minutes after ingestion and can last for up to 12 hours.

As a general rule, experiences can be unpredictable and vary from person to person. Thus, despite their origins, and whether they are natural or artificially produced, the effects of hallucinogens are pretty similar. They can harm one's health if taken in excess.

Chapter 7:

The Future of Dimethyltryptamine

As Dr. Rick Strassman is one of DMT's foremost researchers, he plans to continue his DMT studies at New Mexico's Cottonwood Research Foundation. Meanwhile, Dr. Steven Barker of Louisiana State University is developing an ultra-sensitive way to measure the naturally occurring dimethyltryptamine in the human body. Strassman and Barker seek to compare normal levels with those in altered states under clinical conditions.

Strassman and his team ultimately hope to create a new model of Western consciousness studies. The team hopes to explore the different varieties of human consciousness and their biochemical, psychological, and genetic bases. They hope to find the best way in which to apply these states for reaching greater wisdom, creativity, and healing.

Ayahuasca

Meanwhile, the interest of ayahuasca, which contains DMT, is undoubtedly growing. In an ongoing Global Drug Survey, Adam Winstock, a researcher, and his co-authors determined that DMT "had more new users" as compared to other psychoactive drugs, such as ketamine, LSD, and magic mushrooms.

Winstock's survey's figures are supported by a survey from the National Survey on Drug Use and Health. Both surveys' figures determined that the number of DMT users in the United States has been steadily increasing since 2006 – from around 688,000 during 2006 to 1,475,000 during 2012. The survey also found out that the newest users were more likely to be male, still in school, and young.

The Global Drug Survey, which is held annually, gives a glimpse into how drugs are consumed by users. As the survey does not implement random sampling, it is unable to accurately detect the prevalence of a certain drug's use. However, the survey can identify some of the notable trends.

In an L.A. Weekly report, Los Angeles has at least three ayahuasca subcommittees that are active. On any given night in New York City, there are an estimated 50 to 100 ceremonies that use dimethyltryptamine in ayahuasca.

Around the turn of the millennium, people who were not able to find "acid" in their hometowns started flying to Brazil, Ecuador, or Peru. They hope to experience the still relatively unknown ayahuasca experience. In an interview for the book *This is Your Country on Drugs*, a Peruvian shaman (who sought anonymity) said that before 2001 he never saw an American visit his ceremonies.

Psychedelic Tourism

This form of psychedelic tourism quickly became popular and ayahuasca tours are now offered in South American countries that have no cultural or ceremonial tradition of utilizing the brew. Tommy Thomas, a Costa Rica-based farmer, also spoke on the trend in *This is Your Country on Drugs*.

Formerly a Washington, D.C-based real estate developer, Thomas moved to Costa Rica more than 20 years ago in order to earn a living growing and cultivating hallucinogenic plants. During that time, his hallucinogenic plants were not lucrative so he switched to growing more traditional crops. However, he noticed an upswing on the trade of hallucinogenic plants beginning in 2005.

An indication that ayahuasca tourism has hit critical proportions is exposure in the media. Outlets like National Geographic have run stories on their writers' South American excursions with vomiting, mosquito-riddled camps, and boat/plane/bus rides. However, there is really no need for Americans to travel to South America to experience an ayahuasca trip.

The unnamed Peruvian shaman brought his ayahuasca brew to countries like India, Italy, and Spain during the 1990s. He did not bring his brew to the United States because he did not think that the people would accept it. Eventually, he encountered a few Americans who convinced him to come to San Francisco. Nowadays, he goes to the United States often, and he adds that there are more cities and towns wanting him to come.

Conclusion

Thank you for reading this! We hope this short, concise book was able to teach you a thing or two about DMT.

Now that you understand the important factors regarding DMT, you can decide if you want to try it, or if you can inform your friends who ask you about it. Plus, a little addition to your knowledge doesn't hurt, right? Our world is becoming increasingly interested in the use of DMT and other psychedelic substances, in hopes to enhance the human experience on Earth.

If you've learned anything from this book, please take the time to share your thoughts by sending me a personal message, or even posting a review on Amazon. It would be greatly appreciated and I try my best to get back to every message!

Thank you and good luck in your journey!